WATCH, FIGHT AND PRAY

WATCH FIGHT & PRAY

My Personal Three-fold Strategy
to Combat Prostate Cancer

Lonnell E. Johnson, Ph.D.

Jubilee. PRESS ™
an imprint of Imagine! Books™ • Columbus Ohio

Watch, Fight and Pray: My Personal Three-fold Strategy to Combat Prostate Cancer

Published by Jubilee! Press™, an imprint of Imagine! Books™
part of Imagine! Studios™
P. O. Box 547, Galloway, Ohio 43119
Email: contact@imaginestudiosonline.com
www.imaginestudiosonline.com

Published in Association with Ambassador Press, LLC
P. O. Box 722, Reynoldsburg, Ohio 43068-0722
Email: info@ambassadorpressllc.com
http://ambassadorpressllc.com

All scripture quotations, unless otherwise indicated, are taken from the *Holy Bible, New King James Version®*. Copyright © 1982 by Thomas Nelson, Inc. Used by permission. All rights reserved.

Scripture quotations marked (King James Version) are taken from the *Holy Bible, King James Version*

ISBN 0-9764353-9-X

First Jubilee! Press paperback printing: March 2005

Final Victory

I Corinthians 15:53–57 & Romans 8:37–39

Old man crab is mighty sneaky,
    always creepin and up to no good,
Old man crab, is mighty sneaky,
    always creepin and up to no good,
That low-down dirty rascal,
    Messin with folk all round the neighborhood.

One dark day old man crab came callin,
    Crawlin in like some uninvited mouse,
One dark day old man crab came callin,
    Crawlin in like some uninvited mouse,
That nasty dirty devil,
    Sneakin in the back door of my sister's house.

First you first attacked my mama, old man crab,
    You tried to pinch her with your greatest fears,
First you first attacked my mama, old man crab,
    You tried to pinch her with your greatest fears,
But she didn't want no she-crab soup,
    You tried to served with pain and bitter tears.

You may have come to our house, old man crab,
    But I'm sorry, you can't stay.
You may have come to our house, old man crab,
    But I'm sorry, you can't stay.
Whatsonever in the world you may do,
    Everyday we still gonna watch, fight, and pray.

Nothin' low down on earth, old man crab,
    Or nothin high up in heaven above,
Nothin' low down on earth, old man crab,
    Or nothin high up in heaven above,
Not even death, your creepin pardner,
    Can ever separate us from God's love.

So git out my face, old man crab,
    I got your number, don't you see.
So git out my face, old man crab,
    I got your number, don't you see.
You may win this li'l biddy battle,
    But we show-nuff got the final victory.

Some say our Savior's comin in the mornin;
    Some say in the midnight hour or high noon
Some say our Savior's comin in the mornin;
    Some say in the midnight hour or high noon
I got a feelin He's comin back
    To gather us together soon . . . and very soon.

From *Stone upon Stone: Psalms of Remembrance* ©2001

"Final Victory", an original blues poem, speaks of "Old Man Crab", referring to cancer, the dreaded disease that takes its name from the constellation Cancer, portrayed as "the crab." I was first inspired to compose the poem after the death of my father, Lonnie Johnson, who died of complications from cancer in 1996. My mother, Jessie Marie Johnson, survived two bouts with "Old Man Crab" and after another valiant fight, died of cancer in 2002. I make reference to her first two triumphant battles against cancer in the third stanza. I revised the poem in 2001 after my brother-in-law, Elliott Thompson, passed away from liver cancer. The next year, I was diagnosed with prostate cancer, and the entire poem took on even greater significance, especially this stanza:

> You may have come to our house, old man crab,
>   But I'm sorry, you can't stay.
> You may have come to our house, old man crab,
>   But I'm sorry, you can't stay.
> Whatsonever in the world you may do,
>   Everyday we still gonna watch, fight and pray.

In 2001 after my annual physical examination revealed that my PSA (prostate-specific antigen—a blood factor used to assess the state of the prostate gland) had increased, my physician recommended that I see a urologist. After consultation, he took a biopsy of the prostate which revealed that I had a small amount of cancer in the core of the gland. He explained my options, one of which was to surgically remove the entire gland. I was surprised when he asked if I wanted to schedule the surgery right away. I told him that I wanted to pray about the matter before making a decision and that I would get back with him to let him know my decision.

In the meantime, I informed my wife, Brenda, of the doctor's advice and determined that I would trust God to be healed. I met with my Pastor, Eric Warren, my trusted friend and brother-in-law, and we prayed together. We both "touched and agreed" that God would intervene in the situation and that I would be healed. As we departed, I smiled and said, "Maybe Christ will return, and I won't have to worry about it, after all." That too was another possibility to consider, as I pondered what I would tell the urologist.

Quite providentially my brother-in-law gave me a copy of a newsletter discussing prostate cancer and its treatment from a naturopathic perspective. After reading the newsletter, I began to gather information from a variety of sources, including Larry Burkett's book *Hope for the Hurting*, a most helpful resource which I had given to my sister and her husband when I learned of Elliott's diagnosis. I decided to adopt a posture of "watchful waiting," monitoring my PSA every six months instead of yearly. Prostate cancer is slow growing initially, but it can become more aggressive in later stages and can metastasize to the bone or other organs. I also determined to modify my diet and eliminate red meat and other foods that could possibly contribute to the growth of the cancer. In addition I began to take combination of herbs: saw palmetto and pygeum, along with other vitamins, minerals and supplements.

When I returned to talk with the urologist, I informed him that I would be trying a nutritional approach and that I would be following "watchful waiting" and would not be employing any of the other alternatives. He did not place much credence in herbs and non-traditional approaches, and abruptly ended the discussion by saying for me call him if I changed my mind.

After a period of time, I found a new family physician who also observed an increase in my PSA level, and he likewise advised me to see a urologist to get a second opinion. The new urologist confirmed the diagnosis and explained the options, as the first one had. I informed him that I would continue a position of "watchful waiting." He gave me his card, and suggested that I call him if I needed him. After several months, I called to schedule my semi-annual check-up and PSA blood work, and I discovered that my doctor had relocated to Alaska. I made arrangements to be examined by his replacement, whom I informed of the situation regarding my prostate. My PSA count had increased slightly, from 8.4 to 10.3. This would be considered high but moderately high, and my new doctor expressed some concern and recommended that I make an appointment with the urologist with whom I had last consulted.

Quite providentially, our church was observing a period called Seven Days of Stillness, an exercise designed to bring Christian believers into a closer relationship with God through prayer, specific readings from the Bible, and other activities organized by Chuck Pierce of Glory of Zion International Ministries. I decided to observe the Seven Days of Stillness, as I sought the Lord regarding a strategy to address the situation with my increasing PSA count. During this time God assured me that I was not to panic nor become alarmed and do something rash. "Be still and know that I am God," so the Psalmist declares and so I followed suit with a confident heart at peace with God who has expressed His love to me in so many ways.

Out of this period of reflection and prayer came a strategy to address the condition of my prostate. The poem "Final Victory" provides part of the inspiration for this three-pronged approach to confronting the cancer diagnosis: "To watch, fight and pray." I base this strategy on the foundation of knowing that God loves me, and that nothing can separate me from His endless love, not even death which is mentioned first in Romans 8:37–39 in the list of situations that can never come between us and our Father's love. I poetically express that profound truth in this way:

> Nothin' low down on earth, old man crab,
>> Or nothin high up in heaven above,
> Nothin' low down on earth, old man crab,
>> Or nothin high up in heaven above,
> Not even death, your creepin pardner,
>> Can ever separate us from God's love.

What follows is my personal three-fold strategy to combat prostate cancer: "Watch, Fight and Pray."

WATCH

Jesus exhorts the disciples in Matthew 26:41: "Watch and pray, lest you enter not into temptation. The spirit indeed is willing, but the flesh is weak." To "watch and pray" is a familiar exhortation from the Gospels. With regard to Jesus Christ's return, he also tells his disciples in Mark 13:33: "Take heed, watch and pray; for you do not know when the time is." He goes on to encourage them regarding the same topic in Luke 21:36: "Watch therefore, and pray always that you may be counted worthy to escape all these things that will come to pass, and to stand before the Son of Man."

In the letters written by Paul we find a similar combination of these two verbs. In Colossians 4:2: "Continue earnestly in prayer, and watch in the same with thanksgiving;"[King James Version]. At the end of I Corinthians 16, Paul reminds us in verse 13: "Watch, stand fast in the faith, be brave, be strong."

In I Thessalonians after the comforting words regarding Christ's return in Chapter 5, verses 6–8, Paul goes on to encourage the believers with these words:

> Therefore let us not sleep, as do others; but let us watch and be sober.
> For those who sleep, sleep at night, and those who get drunk are drunk at night.
> But let us, who are of the day, be sober, putting on the breastplate of faith and love, and as a helmet, the hope of salvation.

Paul offers encouragement to Timothy at the end of Paul's final letter to his beloved son in the Gospel:

> II Timothy 4:5
>
> But you be watchful in all things, endure afflictions, do the work of an evangelist, fulfill your ministry.

This final reminder comes from I Peter 4:7 "But the end of all things is at hand: therefore be serious and watchful in your prayers."

"WATCHFUL WAITING"

My specific response to the initial diagnosis of cancer was that of "watchful waiting." Since prostate cancer generally grows slowly, one can elect to undergo none of the more radical treatment alternatives, such as prostatectomy or surgically removing the prostate gland which can result in incontinence and/or impotence. Other alternatives would be radiation therapy or cryotherapy, freezing the prostate and then removing it or one can simply monitor the PSA levels and have a physical examination of the prostate on a more regular basis. I thought of one of the stanzas from one of my favorite hymns, "Blessed Assurance" which captures the essence of this approach for me:

Watching and waiting, looking above,
Filled with His goodness, lost in His love.

FIGHT

In I Timothy 6:12 Paul speaks these words:

> Fight the good fight of faith, lay hold on eternal life, to which you
> were also called and have confessed a good confession in the presence
> of many witnesses.

In preparing to "fight the good fight" I began reading more
extensively on prostate cancer and looking at a variety of alternative
treatments. I purchased a copy of Dr. Don Colbert's book *Bible Cures
for Prostate Disorders.* Among the books he cites is *Dr. Patrick Walsh's
Guide to Surviving Prostate Cancer,* a copy of which I obtained from the
library. In addition I found a number of sources on the internet, one of
which offered a nutritional regimen to lower PSA levels and prevent
metastases of the cancer.

Although I had previously made modifications in my diet, such
as eliminating all red meat, decreasing saturated fats, and eliminating
sugar, there is more that I could do. I had also been taking a saw
palmetto combination, along with other vitamins and minerals, but
there was, likewise, more to be done in this area. My wife and I had
been drinking bottled water for the past two years or so, but there
are other mineral waters that could also facilitate the lowering of
my PSA back down to the normal range. I decided to continue this
approach, but I modified my initial strategy to become more aggressive

in treating the cancer via nutritional means. In exploring alternative treatments, I discovered an extensive Prostate Cancer Protocol offered by Nutrition 2000.

It so happened that this treatment was to be administered for forty days. The number forty is significant in that it symbolically represents a period of testing or trial or probation, as when Jesus was tempted by the devil after being in the wilderness for forty days and nights. This forty-day protocol involved a variety of herbal compounds, vitamins, minerals and dietary adaptations designed to lower the PSA level in men. After the 40 days, patients are encouraged to have their PSA checked, and it should be noticeably lower. This highly involved process seemed ideally suited to me for a number of reasons.

As a former registered pharmacist, licensed in Indiana and North Carolina, I had worked in hospitals most of my pharmacy career spanning more than twenty years. One of the principal compounds was PC Hope, a combination of various herbs and other ingredients. To start the program, the contents of two capsules were to be emptied into two ounces of tomato juice and mixed before drinking. The medication did not mix well with the tomato juice at all. To produce a more palatable mixture, I went back to my training as a pharmacist and developed a formula for an emulsion, using olive oil and bentonite, a natural clay, that I compounded in a two-ounce jar filled with tomato juice.

The entire regimen of mixing and measuring brought to mind fond recollections of days of working full-time as a pharmacist or an apothecary. The entire situation brought to mind another of my poems:

After the Art of the Apothecary

And thou shalt make it an oil of holy ointment,
an ointment compound after the art of the apothecary:
it shall be an holy anointing oil.

Exodus 30:25 [King James Version]

I desire to follow recipes and not to vary
From the prescribed formulas for the remedies I need,
To compound after the art of the apothecary.

I long to work circumspectly and always be wary,
To measure and mix precisely for love and not for greed.
I desire to follow recipes and not to vary.

I recall yearning to learn from childhood days in Gary,
To weigh my decisions and follow as the Lord would lead,
To compound after the art of the apothecary.

I seek to formulate my ideal art and to marry
Vocation and avocation as one of love and need.
I desire to follow recipes and not to vary.

I attempt to move with wisdom but never to tarry
To master each prescription, to excel and to succeed,
To compound after the art of the apothecary.

The sweet smelling savor I desire my life to carry
Is the pure, holy anointing oil tempered of my need.
I desire to follow recipes and not to vary,
To compound after the art of the apothecary.

Fortunately I was on leave of absence from my position as Professor of English at Otterbein College to start a desktop publishing business, Ambassador Press, publisher of this book and others. This new endeavor allowed me the flexibility to carry out the demands of the protocol in terms of time and the demands for consistency in taking the medication. The Nutrition 2000 Prostate Protocol was my attempt to even more aggressively combat the prostate cancer, as I developed the second phase of my strategy.

On the label of some of the dietary supplements were these words:

Jehovah Raphe

I will put none of these diseases on you.
For I, the Lord, am your healer.

This reference from Exodus 15:26 calls to mind one of the redemptive names of God: *Jehovah Rapha, "the Lord, who heals you."* Recalling those words was very comforting and encouraging to me, as I completed the prostate protocol.

As I was concluding this section, I happened to think of other scriptures related to fight, and the passage from Exodus where the Children of Israel confront the Red Sea in their escape from Egypt came to mind:

Exodus 14:14

The LORD will fight for you, and you shall hold your peace.

A similar exhortation came from Deuteronomy 20:4

For the LORD your God is He who goes with you, to fight for you against your enemies, to save you.

There was wonderful encouragement from David who calls to our attention:

Psalm 144:1–2

Blessed be the LORD my Rock,
Who trains my hands for war,
And my fingers for battle—
My lovingkindness and my fortress, My high tower and my deliverer,
My shield, and *the One* in whom I take refuge,
Who subdues my people under me.

With the completion of the Olympic Games during the summer of 2004, I thought of a reference to "fight" from one of my most cherished passages, the athletic analogy from I Corinthians 9:24–27.

Do you not know that those who run in a race all run, but one receives the prize? Run in such a way that you may obtain *it*.

And everyone who competes *for the prize* is temperate in all things. Now they *do it* to obtain a perishable crown, but we *for* an imperishable *crown*.

Therefore I run thus: not with uncertainty. Thus I fight: not as *one who* beats the air.

But I discipline my body and bring *it* into subjection, lest, when I have preached to others, I myself should become disqualified.

The fight we are in is real, and we are not just "shadow-boxing." We must, however, "endure a great fight of afflictions" as mentioned in Hebrews. We have already won, but we just need to finish the course. Then we will be able to say along with Paul:

II Timothy 4:7–8:

I have fought the good fight, I have finished the race, I have kept
the faith: Finally, there is laid up for me the crown of righteousness,
which the Lord, the righteous judge, will give to me on that Day: and
not to me only but also all who have loved His appearing.

THE REAL BATTLEFIELD IS THE MIND

In the arena of spiritual warfare, the real battlefield is the mind. This message is most clearly and concisely expressed in II Corinthians 10:3–5:

> For though we walk in the flesh, we do not war according to the flesh. For the weapons of our warfare are not carnal but mighty in God for pulling down strongholds, Casting down arguments and every high thing that exalts itself against the knowledge of God, bringing every thought into captivity to the obedience of Christ,

In verse 5, "casting down" is *kathaireo*—meaning "to take down (as from a higher place) with the idea of force to pull down, demolish, while "arguments" is a variation of the same verb *kathairesis*, meaning "demolition, extinction—destruction, pulling down."

Without question "renewing the mind" or changing one's thought patterns is an active, aggressive process, as one must seize control of one's thoughts and emotions. Never was I more aware of the importance of controlling my thoughts by putting on the mind of Christ, dispelling the negative thoughts that defeat the promises of God. During the time of the prostate protocol, I was also listening to a teaching series by the renowned Bible teacher, Dr. David Jeremiah, called "Slaying the Giants in Your Life." For each of the giants Dr. Jeremiah discussed, I thought of each one as a personal Goliath, for

whom each individual "David" could defeat with "one smooth stone."
As it turns out, Dr. Jeremiah cited twelve giants, and I supplemented
the teaching with the corresponding opposing emotion to defeat the
giant:

Fear [Love]
Discouragement [Encouragement]
Loneliness [Communion, Fellowship]
Worry [Contentment]
Guilt [Innocence]
Temptation [Responding with the Word: "It is written"]
Anger [Peace]
Resentment [Forgiveness]
Doubt [Faith}
Procrastination [Action]
Failure [Success]
Jealousy [Admiration]

Whenever a believer is confronted with a negative emotion, one
way to overcome this challenge is to move in the opposite direction
with a positive emotion. Perhaps the most difficult emotion to
overcome for me was fear. Because both of my parents were diagnosed
with cancer, in my mind I wrestled with thoughts of accepting the
same condition as inevitable. When I first received the results of the
biopsy, I became involved in an intense internal dialogue in which I
asked myself repeatedly, "What has changed?" My circumstances may
have changed with the diagnosis, but God's love is still the constant
of my life. He cannot love me any more than He does, and He will
not love me any less. I recited in my mind the passage from Romans 8
verse 26 until the end of the chapter. I recognized that according to I
John 4:18 perfect love casts out fear, as I acknowledged that God loved
me and that I loved Him.

That particular teaching series on "Slaying the Giants in Your Life" also corresponded to Chuck Pierce's admonition that we must overcome dangerous emotions, if we are to move into the next season of glory and success.

I listened to another tape by Chuck Pierce during this same period of time, and the statement he made inspired this poem:

Dangerous Emotions

". . . we must overcome our dangerous emotions."

Chuck Pierce

As champions of God, ministers of the Word,
We must overcome each dangerous emotion.
As we fight the good fight, using our shield and sword,
Clothed with the whole armor, not seeking promotion
Of ourselves but of the Savior, who gave His life,
An example that we should follow in His steps,
That we might slay giants of fear, envy and strife.
Stubborn rebellion that would defy God's precepts
And defile desire to serve Him in purity,
We defeat with a smooth stone of obedience.
Resentment, guilt, anger and green-eyed jealousy:
Each deadly emotion yields deadly consequence.
Pride, described as the most dangerous of them all,
Leads to destruction and goes before a downfall.

The process of renewing the mind is ongoing, as each day becomes a challenge to "put off the old man"—those old negative thinking patterns and to put on the new man"—those positive thoughts based on the Word of God. This concept is also referred to as putting on the mind of Christ, and each individual rises to success or failure in the battlefield of the mind.

THE BLOOD OF JESUS CHRIST: A "POWER-FULL" WEAPON

In 2002 on Good Friday, I was privileged to teach the Word of God at our church. I entitled the message "Passover: I Plead the Blood." The focus of the discussion was "the blood of lamb" and its significance both in terms of the Passover and in the crucifixion of Jesus Christ, who is referred to as "our Passover." One of the old hymns I recall from my childhood proclaims "There is power, wonder-working power in the precious blood of the Lamb." I also concentrated on the reality that Jesus Christ bled seven times, as he endured the crucifixion, and I touched upon the expression "to plead the blood." In defining the term, I made this statement:

> Pleading the blood is applying the blood of Jesus Christ to our lives and circumstances, as the Israelites applied the blood of the Passover lamb to their door posts, and they were protected from the destroyer... in the same way we apply the blood to our lives and to circumstances, whereby we need deliverance, whereby we will not be destroyed. 'I plead the blood' expresses the faith in the protective power of the blood of Jesus Christ.

One of the key scriptures I shared was the following:

Revelation 12:11

And they overcame him by the blood of the Lamb and by the word of their testimony, and they did not love their lives to the death.

During this time of healing, certain verses took on a deeper meaning for me as I applied them to my life. This verse from Revelation was one such scripture that came alive for me in a new way.

I also shared the lyrics to a song that I had composed entitled "I Plead the Blood," and at the end of the teaching I led the congregation in making a number of declarations, "pleading the blood" over our congregation, individually, corporately and beyond our geographic location. During my time of healing in the forty-day regimen, I read and sang these words many times:

I plead the blood. I plead the blood.
I plead the blood over my life.
Jesus bled seven times and shed His blood for me
That I might triumph and walk forth in perfected victory.
I plead the blood.

I plead the blood.
I plead the blood.
I plead the blood over my life.

I also listened to that particular teaching tape a number of times, and it ministered to me greatly. Throughout my time of "great distress" I felt like David, who also "encouraged himself in the Lord his God."

Quite providentially I had purchased a booklet by my longtime friend and fellow brother in Christ, Dr. Dale M. Sides, called **40 Days of Communion in Your Home.** Since my prostate treatment involved forty days, I chose to partake of Communion at the end of each day of the protocol. The book discusses various dimensions of the covenant of Holy Communion, one of the avenues for physical and emotional healing. For each day, Dr. Sides offers a scripture and a devotional discussion regarding the New Covenant instituted by Jesus Christ before his crucifixion and resurrection. This daily practice turned out to be another weapon in my arsenal.

PRAY

I keep a prayer journal/scrapbook in which I keep scriptures, poems, song lyrics, quotations, personal prophetic words, photographs, maps and other items that I use daily as touchstones in my time of prayer. Among the scriptures relating to prayer are I Thessalonians 5:17, 18, 25:

> Pray without ceasing. In everything give thanks, for this is the will of God in Christ Jesus for you.

> Brethren, pray for us.

Luke 18:1b reminds us that "...Men ought always to pray and not lose heart." II Thessalonians 3:1–6 offers this powerful exhortation:

> Finally, brethren, pray for us, that the word of the Lord may run *swiftly* and be glorified, just as *it is* with you,

> And that we may be delivered from unreasonable and wicked men; for not all have faith.

> But the Lord is faithful, who will establish you and guard *you* from the evil one.

And we have confidence in the Lord concerning you, both that you do and will do the things we command you.

Now may the Lord direct your hearts into the love of God and into the patience of Christ.

These scriptures are all related to prayer, and most of them are part of my prayer journal/scrapbook. One of the statements I have made regarding prayer is this: "There is always something to pray about." My diagnosis was one more item on my ongoing list of things to pray about or as Pastor Jean Oscar Njock Bayiha, my friend from Senegal, calls them, "prayer topics."

When some of the ministers of our church first started getting together on Saturday mornings, Pastor Luther Henley, one of our pastors, discussed a concept presented by Graham Cooke called "crafting a prayer" from the Scriptures and custom-fitting it to the particular situation for which you are praying. I thought of crafting a prayer for my cancer diagnosis when I realized that, indeed, I already had crafted such a prayer.

Last year at our church I prepared a teaching based on the statement made by my sister, Cheryl Thompson, in response to being in an undesirable situation. She commented that God is doing one or a combination of things when we find ourselves in the midst of a "fiery trial": He is endeavoring to "Direct you, Inspect you, Correct you, Protect you, or Perfect you." That statement I transformed into a teaching "A Five-Fold Prayer: Direct Me, Inspect Me, Correct Me, Protect Me, Perfect Me."

In the message I discussed each of the five verbs, using scriptures, anecdotes and personal incidents as well as related music. Each section concluded with a poem, a psalm expressing my desire to God with regard to that particular verb. I thought of the section "Protect Me" as closely related to my present situation. Since the word "protect" is not found in the King James Version, which I most often use, I thought of using the word "deliver" instead.

In the Old Testament the verb "deliver" means "to pluck out of the hands of an oppressor or enemy; to preserve, recover, remove; to deliver from danger, evil, trouble; to be delivered, to escape." Psalm 31:1–5 is especially encouraging:

> In You, O Lord, I put my trust;
> Let me never be ashamed;
> Deliver me in Your righteousness.
> Bow down Your ear to me,
> Deliver me speedily;
> Be my rock of refuge,
> A fortress of defense to save me.
> For You *are* my rock and my fortress;
> Therefore, for Your name's sake,
> Lead me and guide me.
> Pull me out of the net which they have secretly laid for me,
> For You *are* my strength.
> Into Your hand I commit my spirit;
> You have redeemed me, O Lord God of truth.

In the New Testament the word "deliver" is translated from *ruomai* which means "to draw or snatch to one's self from danger, to rescue, to deliver." In the poem "Why Don't Somebody Help Me Praise the Lord?" I relate that God personally intervened in my life and rescued or delivered me:

> With loving arms you reached way down
> And snatched me from Satan's outhouse,
> Sought me and flat-out rescued me,
> Fixed me up in my Father's house.
> *"Why Don't Somebody Help Me Praise the Lord?"*

In John 17:15 Jesus Christ makes this statement to God, His Father: "I do not pray that You should take them out of the world, but that You should keep them from the evil one."

Matthew 6:13 provides a similar kind of request expressed in what has become known as "The Lord's Prayer":

> And do not lead us not into temptation,
> But deliver us from the evil one:
> For Yours is the kingdom and the power and the glory for ever.
> Amen.

II Thessalonians 3:3 offers this reminder:

> But the Lord is faithful, who shall establish you, and guard you from the evil one.

II Timothy 4:18 makes a similar declaration:

> And the Lord will deliver me from every evil work and preserve me for His heavenly kingdom. To Him be glory forever and ever. Amen!

This section of the teaching concludes with a prayer:

> As a child runs to safety in his father's arms,
> So I, too, run to you, "my shelter from life's storms."
> Lord, I long to dwell with you in the secret place,
> My buckler, my shield, deliverer, my fortress,
> Strong tower, defender, who responds to my prayer.
> For Lord, you are faithful, who will establish me
> And protect me and deliver me from evil.

This particular section of the teaching seemed perfectly "crafted" to my situation regarding the diagnosis of prostate cancer and the elevated PSA level. I thought of augmenting it, however, when I recalled a passage from II Corinthians 1:9–10 which I added to my arsenal in this area of spiritual warfare:

> Yes, we had the sentence of death in ourselves, that we should not trust in ourselves but in God who raises the dead,

> Who delivered us from so great a death, and does deliver us: in whom we trust that He will still deliver us;

I realized that the diagnosis of cancer can be seen by some as a "death sentence", but the exhortation is not to trust in ourselves but in God who raises the dead, should the death sentence be actually carried out, as it will be one way or another, should the Lord tarry. In actuality sin is the death sentence which is manifested, not only in cancer but in a whole range of deadly diseases; indeed, the wages of sin is death. Despite this diagnosis, I continued to trust God, that just as He has delivered those who trusted Him in the past and is presently delivering those who continue to trust Him, so will He yet continue to deliver in the future. I rejoiced as I added those verses to the end of the "Protect Me" section of my "crafted prayer."

PRAYING IN THE SPIRIT— POWER OF PERFECT PRAYER

In the First Epistle to the Corinthians, Paul relates two ways to pray to God: to "pray with the spirit" and to "pray with the understanding." To pray "with the understanding," is to pray in the language that one normally speaks, as if you were having a conversation with God. To "pray in the spirit is to pray in tongues or to pray in an unknown language to you the speaker, in the tongue of men or of angels, as mentioned in I Corinthians 13:1. Some refer to this spiritual ability as communicating with God in one's "prayer language."

I Corinthians 14:15 makes this statement:

> What is *the conclusion* then? I will pray with the spirit, and I will also pray with the understanding. I will sing with the spirit, and I will sing with the understanding.

In this section of I Corinthians 14 Paul continues discussing "spiritual matters" or "gifts of the spirit," referring to speaking in tongues or "giving thanks well." Some have called this "perfect prayer" or "perfect praise."

Paul concludes the Book of Ephesians with this exhortation:

Ephesians 6:10–18:

Finally, my brethren, be strong in the Lord and in the power of His might.

Put on the whole armor of God, that you may be able to stand against the wiles of the devil.

For we do not wrestle against flesh and blood, but against principalities, against powers, against the rulers of the darkness of this age, against spiritual *hosts* of wickedness in the heavenly *places.*

Therefore take up the whole armor of God, that you may be able to withstand in the evil day, and having done all, to stand.

Stand therefore, having girded your waist with truth, having put on the breastplate of righteousness,

And having shod your feet with the preparation of the gospel of peace;

Above all, taking the shield of faith with which you will be able to quench all the fiery darts of the wicked one.

And take the helmet of salvation, and the sword of the Spirit, which is the word of God;

Praying always with all prayer and supplication in the Spirit, being watchful to this end with all perseverance and supplication for all the saints—

For the Christian believer putting on the whole armor of God should be applicable to every situation, but this passage had particular application to my specific situation regarding cancer, especially the last verse of the passage:

Praying always with all prayer and supplication in the Spirit, being watchful to this end with all perseverance and supplication for all saints—

Verse 20 of Jude also makes this reference to "praying in the Holy Spirit" or in the Holy Ghost:

But you, beloved, building up on your most holy faith, praying in the Holy Spirit.

In Paul's epistle to the Romans, he speaks of praying in the spirit, which bypasses the mind, as a means of expressing that which you can not adequately communicate in words.

Romans 8:26:

Likewise the Spirit also helps our weaknesses: for we know not what we should pray for as we ought: but the Spirit Himself makes intercession for us with groanings which cannot be uttered.

Throughout this period of time following my diagnosis of cancer, there were times when I could not clearly articulate a prayer with my understanding, and so I relied heavily on praying in the spirit in addition to praying with my understanding.

FAITH, THE ESSENTIAL INGREDIENT

"But without faith it is impossible. . . ."

In the beginning of 2004 quite providentially I was asked to teach during a mid-week Bible study when our senior pastor was out of town. He had begun a series on the gifts or manifestations of the spirit from I Corinthians 12, and I was asked to teach on faith. This subject was particularly important to me since it was the topic of the first teaching from the Bible I had ever done back in the late 1950s when I was a sophomore in high school, attending a summer camp in northern Michigan. I volunteered to prepare a little "sermonette" on any subject, and I chose faith. Using the resources of one of the camp counselors who was a seminary student, I looked at Hebrews 11, especially verses 1 and 6:

> Now faith is the substance of things hoped for, the evidence of things not seen.

> But without faith *it is* impossible to please *Him,* for he who comes to God must believe that He is, and *that* He is a rewarder of those who diligently seek Him.

Almost fifty years later I enjoyed reminiscing with our congregation, as we examined the Word of God and pointed out significant illustrations of faith in the Scriptures and in my life. I

34

endeavored to relate the simplicity of faith, being that of hearing from God by way of the written Word or the Bible or by revelation from God. By acting upon what you have heard, you receive the corresponding results of your actions. Romans 10:17 reminds us of the source of faith:

> So then faith comes by hearing and hearing by the word of God.

During the time of my 40-day prostate protocol, I "just happened" to come across the tape of that particular teaching and listened to the tape over and over, in an effort to build my faith.

I also recalled the personal prophecy I received from Dr. Kingsley Fletcher in 2000 regarding the dimension of faith in my life. A personal prophecy or prophetic words are inspired words from an individual operating the gift of prophecy to speak to a specific individual or group. These insightfully penetrating words are revealed from God and provide edification, exhortation and comfort to the individuals to whom they are addressed. On this specific occasion when Dr. Fletcher ministered at our church, he called me forth and spoke a message from God to me. I transcribed those words and added them to my prayer journal/scrapbook. Numerous times I read and re-read those words as I prayed during those forty days. I especially concentrated on this excerpt:

> *The anointing of the Lord is upon you. You shall walk through doors, and you shall bring the people of God behind you. No man shall be able to stand before you all the days of your life. Mighty man of faith! When you declare, it shall be done. You shall affect many through your faith, for out of the faith you shall see my faithfulness. . . . And you shall declare this is the way of the Lord, and they shall follow. For you shall stand and declare just as Caleb declared. You shall stand and say, 'If God said it, it shall come to pass. If God declares it, I believe it. If God points the way, I will follow.'*

And the people of God shall be inspired by your humble faith. For you are a man that has pleased me, and I'm delighted in you. This is the word of the Lord to you, Lonnell. To Lonnell, the word of the Lord. You shall walk in faith and not by sight.

I used that particular prophetic word as a contact point for focused intercession regarding my particular situation with the prostate cancer.

Last year I attended an Apostolic School of Ministry in Pietermaritzburg, South Africa, where I heard a teaching that encapsulated what I had been doing, as I was meditating deeply on the words of my personal prophecy. That teaching inspired this poem which also came to mean a great deal to me during the time of the testing of my faith:

Prophetic Words and Apostolic Charge

This charge I commit to you, son Timothy, according to the prophecies previously made concerning you, that by them you may wage the good warfare,

I Timothy 1:18

As Paul reminded Timothy, his own true son,
To give heed and weigh the words of prophecy
And to accept the apostolic charge he gave,
So we must recall the prophetic registers
That follow our lives and employ prophetic words
As battle axes used in spiritual warfare,
As we craft governmental prayers to reach God's throne.
We look at prophetic words as the Bereans,
Who received the Word with all readiness of mind
And validated that indeed those things were so.
Just as Israel prophesied to each of his sons,
So our prophetic words live beyond our lifetimes.

36

We progressively walk into our destiny
Through prophetic words and our apostolic charge.

At times when my faith seemed to be diminishing, I would recite Scripture, listen to teaching tapes, in many cases my own messages whereby I taught myself over and over again. During this time of intense prayer, God was teaching me a valuable lesson about faith: "Prayer is the key . . . but faith unlocks the door." I was reminded of these lyrics from an old gospel song, as I prayed fervently throughout this situation which seemed to be drawing from within me to become the "mighty man of faith" that God called me to be.

THE END OF FORTY DAYS

"Tell me how did you feel when you come out the wilderness?"

Originally I had scheduled my regular doctor's appointment for three months after my last visit, which would have been in December of 2004. As I completed the protocol, I rescheduled my appointment in order to have my PSA level checked at the end of the forty days. As the day approached for my new appointment, my heart and my mind raced with excitement. As I ended the last phase of my 40-day journey through the wilderness, the lyrics to a number of songs came to mind as I would go through the days. One, in particular, is an old spiritual which asks a question and provides a personal response:

> *Tell me how did you feel when you come out the wilderness?*
> *Come out the wilderness? Come out the wilderness?*
> *Tell me how did you feel when you come out the wilderness?*
> *Leaning on the Lord.*
>
> *I felt like shouting when I come out the wilderness.*
> *. . . come out the wilderness.*
> *. . . come out the wilderness.*
> *I felt like shouting when I come out the wilderness,*
> *Leaning on the Lord.*

The choruses repeat with the verbs: "singing", "dancing", "praising", etc., and I felt all of those responses and more, as the day approached for my appointment.

Another song came to mind as I completed the last official day of the Prostate Protocol, in anticipation of my latest PSA level. From time to time, I have heard an old gospel number by Shirley Caesar "You're Next in Line for A Miracle" in which the choir sings:

> You're next in line for a miracle.
> You have kept the faith. Today is your day for a miracle.
> Take it by faith. . . Take it by faith.
> Today is your day for a miracle.

After a number of delays, such as having to get gas and returning home to get a heavier jacket, I finally arrived at the doctor's office. I signed in, and while I was waiting, a series of informative videos was playing in the waiting room, each discussing various medical conditions and their treatment. As I sat down, a discussion came on regarding the effect of soy products on various conditions, including prostate cancer. I smiled, acknowledging that I had increased my intake of soy nuts, tofu, iso-flavones, and other products containing soy since my initial diagnosis. I see this as a mild confirmation of that particular part of my regimen.

When my doctor arrived, I explained the purpose of my visit was to have my PSA checked. I shared with him the circumstances of my request in light of the 40-day protocol which I had just completed. As I was speaking to him, I observed a light in his eyes and a sympathetic response when I shared that my strategy came during a ten-day period of seeking God. I am certain that he is a Christian, for I recognized that familiar look in the eyes that mirrors the soul of a fellow believer. As the saying goes, "It takes one to know one."

He said he will call me with the results of the blood test when they come back. He also cautioned me that he will be concerned and will recommend that I contact the urologist, should the PSA level go up. I leave rejoicing that "my miracle is on the way."

The next day the doctor called and informed me of the reading: 3.15. From a 10.3 to 3.15—a seven point decrease! My PSA level went from a notably high level to a normal level for a man my age. Although I was not at home when he called, he left the message with my wife, and we rejoiced and celebrated together. So many scriptures came to mind as I acknowledged God's faithfulness. Passages from the Psalms flooded my soul. Psalm 103:1–5 makes this declaration:

> Bless the Lord, O my soul;
> And all that is within me, *bless* His holy name!
> Bless the Lord, O my soul,
> And forget not all His benefits:
> Who forgives all your iniquities,
> Who heals all your diseases,
> Who redeems your life from destruction,
> Who crowns you with lovingkindness and
> tender mercies,
> Who satisfies your mouth with good *things,*
> *So that* your youth is renewed like the eagle's.

I also echo the words of the Psalmist who also states, "I sought the Lord, and he heard me, and delivered me from all my fears." Earlier this week, I rejoiced in Psalm 124:7 which seemed to speak to me in a special way:

> Our soul has escaped as a bird from the snare of the fowlers: the snare is broken, and we have escaped.

I continued to joy and rejoice, as I shared the news that a miracle with my name on it had arrived. In actuality the special delivery package had been had been sent long ago. The reality of the physical healing of my body occurred when God first *thought* it before He *spoke* it and I walked into the actual manifestation. Even before I began the 40-day protocol, I firmly believed that there was "miracle with my name on it." Friday, November 5, 2004 at 5:30 p.m. was the delivery date, but in actuality this particular miracle of healing had been accomplished centuries ago when Jesus Christ shed his blood for the remission of my sins, and by his stripes I was healed. Now I am walking into the physical manifestation of that spiritual accomplishment.

A few years ago on Passover, which coincided with Good Friday, I attended a service at our church. As the Senior Pastor, Eric L. Warren, expounded upon the significance of the feast of Passover, I understood the sacrifice of Jesus Christ in a profoundly deeper way and applied that teaching to my life. I was able to crystallize and personalize that message in a poem:

Taking It Personally

Isaiah 53

Cursed with a curse, He was hung on a tree.
The suffering servant bartered for a price,
Battered and bruised for my iniquity.
Behold the Lamb, unblemished sacrifice,
Offered once, Jesus Christ, my Passover.
Afflicted, stricken, smitten that God should
Freely pour out His mercy, moreover,
Lay on Him the chastisement of my peace.
From His side flowed water and sinless blood,
A new covenant established that I might cease
From dead works by a new and living way.
God's good pleasure no longer concealed

41

But memorialized this solemn day.
    Man of sorrows, with His stripes I am healed
In spirit, mind and body, for I am
    Quickened and cleansed by the blood of the Lamb.

April 15, 1998
Passover

WATCH, FIGHT AND PRAY

This triple threat, a one-two-three combination, was my personal strategy to gain the victory over the physical condition of prostate cancer, but the same plan can be adapted to any challenge—physical, emotion, financial or to whatever is needed. First of all, maintain a watchful attitude. The treacherous times in which we live demand that we "walk circumspectly" (Ephesians 5:15), that is, "watchful on all sides" because the days are evil. Watch what you put into your mouth, and watch what you put into your mind as well. Remember Jesus Christ's exhortation to watch and pray.

Not only are we called to watch, but we are also encouraged to fight the good fight, being ever mindful that we do not wrestle against flesh and blood but that ours is a spiritual battle. Recognize that the real battlefield is the mind. As David ran toward Goliath to defeat that monstrous giant with a single shot from his sling, move forward aggressively as you put off old thinking patterns and put on new ways of thinking, based on the Scriptures. As we renew our minds and put on the whole armor of God, The Lord God of Hosts, our Commander-in-Chief will not only fight for us but will also teach our hands to war. He will give us the winning strategies to defeat every enemy.

Finally we must maintain an attitude of prayer, as we pray without ceasing. Again Christ reminds us that we should always pray and not faint. I am reminded that there is always something to pray about.

One of the most powerful ways of praying is to "pray the Scriptures", that is reciting sections from the Bible as though they were prayers. "Crafting a prayer" is also beneficial, whereby we find specific passages that address the issue at hand and apply those verses to that particular situation.

Like Paul, we can pray in the spirit and pray with our understanding also.

Although prayer is indispensable in the life of a believer, we must do more than offer up our prayers; we must get up and give feet to our prayers by doing the will of God. We must not only be hearers of the Word, but we must be doers as well.

We watch, fight and pray with the full knowledge that Christ defeated the enemy at Calvary, and that in all these things we are more than conquerors. We stand secure in knowing that our times are in God's hands and that as Isaiah 49:16 declares, "See, I have inscribed you on the palms *of My hands;* Your walls *are* continually before Me."

Knowing just how much God loves us, we conclude our three-fold strategy to "Watch, Fight and Pray" with this encouraging and comforting reminder:

Philippians 4:6–7:

Be anxious for nothing; but in everything by prayer and supplication, with thanksgiving, let your requests be made known to God;

And the peace of God, which surpasses all understanding will guard your hearts and minds through Christ Jesus.

ABOUT THE AUTHOR

Described as a "real Renaissance Man," Lonnell E. Johnson, Ph.D. represents a unique collage of experiences as a poet, professor, minister and motivational speaker. He has worked as a pharmacist, information analyst, editor, administrator and director of public relations, as well as university professor. His use of original poetry, his vivid illustrations, and delightful humor also provide a special flavor as motivational and inspirational speaker.

He has written numerous biblical research articles and is author of two collections of poetry *Ears Near to the Lips of God* (1984) and *Sacred Jazz: Music, Mood, and Mind* (1994). Dr. Johnson has captivated audiences across the country with his lively poetry performances with musical accompaniment.

In addition, Professor Johnson has also published scholarly articles in the area of African American Literature. Currently he is on leave of absence from his position as Professor of English at Otterbein College in Westerville, Ohio. Most recently he established Ambassador Press, publishers of *Stone upon Stone: Psalms of Remembrance* (2004) with accompanying CDs of his reading the poems with music. Dr. Johnson also offers his testimony of faith in *Watch, Fight and Pray: My Personal Strategy to Combat Prostate Cancer* (2005).

OTHER RESOURCES BY LONNELL E. JOHNSON

"Good News Day"—Daybreaking Series (CD)

Sacred Jazz: Music, Mood and Mind

Stone upon Stone: Psalms of Remembrance
   Book and CDs

*Watch, Fight and Pray: My Personal Three-fold Strategy
   to Combat Prostate Cancer*

Visit **www.ambassadorpressllc.com** for a complete listing of resources from
Ambassador Press, LLC, P.O. Box 722, Reynoldsburg, OH 43068-0722 or
send an email request to ambpress@insight.rr.com